Table of Contents

INTRODUCTION

You may be able to prevent kidney stones from forming with dietary changes, including staying hydrated, consuming more citrus, and avoiding certain foods like those high in sodium.

Kidney stones in the urinary tract are formed in several ways. Calcium can combine with chemicals, such as oxalate or phosphorous, in the urine. This can happen if these substances become so concentrated that they solidify. Kidney stones can also be caused by a buildup of uric acid. Uric acid buildup is caused by the metabolism of protein.

Your urinary tract wasn't designed to expel solid matter, so it's no surprise that kidney stones are very painful to pass. Luckily, they can usually be avoided through diet.

WHAT IS KIDNEY STONE

A kidney stone diet, also known as a renal stone diet, is a specialized eating plan designed to prevent the formation of kidney stones or manage existing conditions related to kidney stones. Kidney stones are solid masses that form in the kidneys when certain minerals and substances in the urine crystallize and accumulate. They can be painful to pass and can lead to various health complications.

The primary goal of a kidney stone diet is to reduce the risk of developing new stones or assist in managing conditions like hypercalciuria (excessive calcium in the urine), which can contribute to stone formation. The diet typically focuses on maintaining proper fluid intake, reducing the consumption of specific minerals, and promoting a balanced and nutrient-rich diet.

People who wish to prevent kidney stones developing for the first time or reduce the risk of recurrence if they have already had stones should follow these main steps:

Key components of a kidney stone diet include:

1. **Hydration:** Drinking an adequate amount of fluids is essential to prevent kidney stone formation. Water helps dilute urine, making it less likely for minerals to crystallize and form stones. Aim to drink enough water throughout the day.

2. **Low Oxalate Intake:** Foods high in oxalates, such as spinach, rhubarb, beets, and certain nuts, can contribute to calcium oxalate stone formation. Reducing the consumption of these foods may be recommended.

3. **Balanced Calcium Intake:** Contrary to popular belief, adequate calcium intake is important for kidney stone prevention. Calcium binds to

oxalates in the intestines, reducing the risk of them entering the urinary tract. Focus on obtaining calcium from dietary sources or supplements, as advised by a healthcare professional.

4. **Sodium Reduction:** High sodium intake can lead to increased calcium excretion in urine, potentially contributing to stone formation. Reducing salt consumption and avoiding high-sodium processed foods is beneficial.

5. **Limiting Animal Protein:** High intake of animal protein, such as red meat and poultry, can increase the excretion of certain substances that contribute to stone formation. Moderation is key.

6. **Including Fiber:** Consuming adequate dietary fiber can help reduce the risk of kidney stones by promoting regular bowel movements and decreasing calcium absorption.

7. **Monitoring Protein Intake:** Some individuals may benefit from controlling protein intake, as excessive protein can lead to increased excretion of substances that form stones.

It's important to note that a kidney stone diet should be tailored to an individual's specific medical history, type of stones, and underlying health conditions. Consulting a healthcare professional or registered dietitian is crucial before making significant dietary changes to prevent kidney stone formation or manage existing conditions.

There is no single diet plan for all types of kidney stones, as they can form due to a buildup of several different minerals in the body. However, many dietitians and doctors who specialize in kidney diseases, or nephrologists, recommend the Dietary Approaches to Stop Hypertension (DASH) diet for people with kidney stones.

This diet has demonstrated the ability to reduce the risk of kidney stone formation and improve other elements of overall health, such as lower blood pressure and a reduced risk of heart disease, stroke, and cancer.

The DASH diet encourages people to consume vegetables, fruits, whole grains, and low-fat dairy. The plan also suggests limiting the intake of salt, sugar, and red meat.

However, dietary changes mainly affect people at risk of the following types of kidney stone:

- ❖ calcium oxalate stones

- ❖ calcium phosphate stones

- ❖ uric acid stones

- ❖ cystine stones

People should speak with their healthcare provider to work out which type of kidney stones they have had, if any, to support effective dietary choices. The National Kidney Foundation recommend cutting back on sodium in the diet rather than reducing calcium intake.

Are All Kidney Stones The Same?

The most common types of kidney stones are calcium stones followed by uric acid stones. Diet changes and medical treatment are individualized based on the type of stone, to prevent them from coming back.

How Can I Prevent Kidney Stones?

Kidney stones are no fun. But With the right foods, plenty of water, and proper medication, you can lower your chances of getting them.

Risk Factors for Kidney Stones

"Kidney stones" is a term that covers different types of small, solid crystals. They can have different causes and different food culprits. Some are related to kidney infections. Others form because you have too much of certain minerals in your system or not enough of the substances that keep stones from forming.

Genes can play a role, too. Forty percent of the people who get kidney stones have relatives who have them, too. Their bodies may get rid of too much calcium or too little citrate (a chemical found in citrus fruits) in their pee, for instance.

Other conditions that make kidney stones more likely include:

❖ **Obesity**. When you're overweight, you tend to get them more often. The same is true if you have diabetes.

❖ **Gout**. This painful condition happens when uric acid builds up in your blood. That makes crystals form in your joints or kidneys.

❖ **Diabetes**. Insulin resistance from diabetes can raise calcium levels in your urine, making kidney stones more likely.

- ❖ **Intestinal surgery.** If you've had certain types of gastric bypass surgery or other intestinal surgery, your risk may go up.

- ❖ **Hyperparathyroidism**. It can raise calcium levels in your blood and trigger kidney stones.

- ❖ **Certain kidney diseases**. One example is polycystic kidney disease, in which clusters of cysts grow in your kidneys. Another is medullary sponge kidney, a birth defect that causes cysts to form in the organ's tubes.

- ❖ **Middle-aged men** are most likely to get kidney stones, though it can happen to people of any age or sex.

Causes of Kidney Stones

Even if you're in good health, your diet may encourage kidney stones to grow. One top reason is you may not be drinking enough water. That means you'll make too little pee, which gives the stones more chances to form.

Other things to watch:

- ❖ **Colas**. These beverages are high in fructose and phosphates, which may lead to kidney stones.

❖ **Oxalates**. These are organic compounds found in
a number of foods, including healthy ones such as
spinach and sweet potatoes. But oxalates also
bind easily to certain minerals, including calcium,
which then help form kidney stones.

❖ **Salt (specifically, sodium).** Lots of sodium, which
you get mainly through salt. means more calcium
in your pee. That ups your odds for kidney stones.
Eating calcium-rich foods like kale and salmon is
OK unless you also eat too much salt. Too little
calcium in your diet may lead to kidney stones in
certain people.

❖ **Vitamin C supplements.** Be careful with these.
Research has found high doses of vitamin C taken
regularly can double a man's chances for a kidney
stone. There's no need to worry about vitamin C
in food.

❖ **Animal protein.** Too many steaks, chicken, eggs,
and seafood can build up calcium and uric acid in
your body. That's another cause of kidney stones.

❖ **Medications.** Some prescription and over-the-
counter drugs can contribute to kidney stones,
including antacids, certain antibiotics,
decongestants, diuretics, steroids and certain
medicines for cancer, HIV, and epilepsy.

❖ **Previous kidney stones.** If you've had them once, you're likely to get them again, unless you take steps.

What You Can Do to Prevent Kidney Stones

If you've already had a kidney stone, your doctor may recommend medication to keep it from happening again. What kind will depend on what caused the stone.

Also, take charge of your diet:

Drink lots of water. Stay hydrated, especially when you exercise. Aim for at least 80 ounces per day.

Check food labels. Read the ingredients. Avoid or cut back on foods with high amounts of ingredients like sodium chloride, monosodium glutamate (MSG), and sodium nitrate.

Limit meat intake.

Choose foods wisely. Usually it's good to get more spinach and nuts in your diet. But if you have calcium oxalate stones, which are the most common type, your doctor may tell you to avoid or limit foods high in oxalates:

- ❖ Nuts, including almonds, cashews, pistachios, and peanuts

- ❖ Soy products, including soy burgers, soy milk, and soy cheese

- ❖ Chocolate

- ❖ Oat and oat bran

- ❖ Red kidney beans, navy beans, and fava beans

- ❖ Beets, spinach, kale, and tomato

These foods are low in oxalates. Caution: Too much dairy food and animal protein can up your chances of less common types of kidney stones:

- ❖ Grapes, melons, bananas

- ❖ Cucumbers, cauliflower, cabbage, peas

- ❖ Cheese, milk, butter

- ❖ Beef, bacon, chicken, ham

- ❖ Eat citrus fruits. Lemons and limes are high in citrate, which helps prevent kidney stones.

Get plenty of calcium. Not enough calcium in your diet can lead to kidney stones. It's better if you get it from food, like low-fat dairy products, rather than supplements.

Doctors break down kidney stones into types. Knowing which kind you have could affect the treatment you get. They include:

❖ Calcium stones: These are the most common ones. Even just eating some foods very high in oxalates, such as rhubarb, or taking unusually high levels of vitamin D, can boost your chances of getting this type. You could get this kind if you typically don't drink enough water or if you sweat a lot and don't replace the fluids you lose.

❖ Cystine stones: This is the least common type and due to a genetic mutation. In this situation, your kidneys have trouble reabsorbing a compound called cystine, which ends up in the urine at higher levels and causes stones to form.

❖ Struvite stones: Infections, especially in the urinary tract, can cause this kind of stone.

❖ Uric acid stones: Eating large amounts of animal proteins can lead to uric acid buildup in your urine. That can eventually form a stone either with or without calcium. Risk factors include gout, diabetes, and chronic diarrhea.

How does your doctor know if you really do have a kidney stone? First, they'll get a medical history and examine you. Then, if needed, they'll order tests to get pictures of your kidneys and urinary tract.

You might get:

- ❖ **Blood tests:** They can show if you have too much calcium or uric acid in your blood. They also tell your doctor a lot about how healthy your kidneys are.

- ❖ **Urine test:** The doctor may tell you to collect one or two 24-hour samples. It shows if there are too many stone-forming minerals in your urine or not enough of other compounds that stop stones from forming.

- ❖ **Imaging tests:** Doctors use these to check for stones in your urinary tract. You might get an X-ray of your belly or a computerized tomography (CT) scan, which combines a series of X-rays to make a picture of your body. An X-ray can show larger stones, but the CT scan helps doctors find small ones.

- ❖ **Analysis of passed stones:** The doctor will get you to pee through a strainer to catch any stones you might pass. They'll send them to a lab to see what they're made of. This can tell them what's causing your stones and how to treat them.

❖ Pregnant women should get an ultrasound rather than a CT scan in the first trimester, when babies are most at risk of a radiation injury. A low-dose CT scan is less dangerous in the second and third trimesters.

When to call a doctor

If you're in really bad pain, you'll probably want to see a doctor. Other signs you should quickly seek medical care include:

❖ Being sick to your stomach and throwing up while in pain

❖ Being feverish and cold off and on while in pain

❖ Having bloody urine or a hard time going

Diet Recommendations for Kidney Stones

General Recommendations

Drink plenty of fluid: 2-3 quarts/day

This includes any type of fluid such as water, coffee and lemonade which have been shown to have a beneficial effect with the exception of grapefruit juice and soda.

This will help produce less concentrated urine and ensure a good urine volume of at least 2.5L/day

- ❖ Limit foods with high oxalate content

- ❖ Spinach, many berries, chocolate, wheat bran, nuts, beets, tea and rhubarb should be eliminated from your diet intake

- ❖ Eat enough dietary calcium

- ❖ Three servings of dairy per day will help lower the risk of calcium stone formation. Eat with meals.

- ❖ Avoid extra calcium supplements

- ❖ Calcium supplements should be individualized by your physician and registered kidney dietitian

- ❖ Eat a moderate amount of protein

- ❖ High protein intakes will cause the kidneys to excrete more calcium therefore this may cause more stones to form in the kidney

- ❖ Avoid high salt intake

- ❖ High sodium intake increases calcium in the urine which increases the chances of developing stones

- ❖ Low salt diet is also important to control blood pressure.

- ❖ Avoid high doses of vitamin C supplements

It is recommend to take 60mg/day of vitamin C based on the US Dietary Reference Intake

Excess amounts of 1000mg/day or more may produce more oxalate in the body

What to eat and drink

If you're trying to avoid kidney stones, what you eat and drink is as important as what you shouldn't eat and drink. Here are some important rules of thumb to keep in mind.

- ❖ Stay hydrated

Fluids, especially water, help to dilute the chemicals that form stones. Try to drink at least 12 glasses of water a day.

- ❖ Up your citrus intake

Citrus fruit, and their juice, can help reduce or block the formation of stones due to naturally occurring citrate. Good sources of citrus include lemons, oranges, and grapefruit.

❖ Eat lots of calcium (and vitamin D)

If your calcium intake is low, oxalate levels may rise. It's preferable to get your calcium from food, rather than from supplements, as these have been linked to kidney stone formation. Good sources of calcium include milk, yogurt, cottage cheese, and other types of cheeses. Vegetarian sources of calcium include legumes, calcium-set tofu, dark green vegetables, nuts, seeds, and blackstrap molasses. If you don't like the taste of cow's milk, or, if it doesn't agree with you, try lactose-free milk, fortified soy milk, or goat's milk. Also make sure to include foods high in vitamin D each day. Vitamin D helps the body absorb more calcium. Many foods are fortified with this vitamin. It's also found in fatty fishes, such as salmon, mushrooms, and cheese.

Food and drinks to avoid on a kidney stone diet

❖ Limit salt

High sodium levels in the body, can promote calcium buildup in urine. Avoid adding salt to food, and check the labels on processed foods to see how much sodium they contain. Fast food can be high in sodium, but so can regular restaurant food. When you're able, ask that no salt be added to whatever you order on a menu. Also, take note of what you drink. Some vegetable juices are high in sodium.

❖ Lower your animal protein intake

Many sources of protein, such as red meat, pork, chicken, poultry, and eggs, increase the amount of uric acid you produce. Eating large amounts of protein also reduces a chemical in urine called citrate. Citrate's job is to prevent the formation of kidney stones. Alternatives to animal protein include quinoa, tofu (bean curd), hummus, chia seeds, and Greek yogurt. Since protein is important for overall health, discuss how much you should eat daily with your doctor.

❖ Be mindful of oxalates

Eat oxalates wisely. Foods high in this chemical may increase formation of kidney stones. If you've already had kidney stones, you may wish to reduce or eliminate oxalates from your diet completely. If you're trying to avoid kidney stones, check with your doctor to determine if limiting these foods is enough. If you do eat foods containing oxalates, always make sure to eat or drink a calcium source with them. This will help the oxalate bind to the calcium during digestion, before it can reach your kidneys. Foods high in oxalate include:

- chocolate

- beets

- nuts

- tea

- rhubarb

- spinach

- swiss chard

- sweet potatoes

- Don't drink colas

Avoid cola drinks. Cola is high in phosphate, another chemical which can promote the formation of kidney stones.

❖ Reduce or eliminate added sugar intake

Added sugars are sugars and syrups that are added to processed foods and drinks. Added sucrose and added fructose may increase your risk of kidney stones. Keep an eye on the amount of sugar you eat, in processed foods, such as cake, in fruit, in soft drinks, and in juices. Other common added sugar names include corn syrup, crystallized fructose, honey, agave nectar, brown rice syrup, and cane sugar.

How does the diet work?

Some foods contain certain chemicals or compounds that can influence the production of kidney stones, particularly if a person regularly eats them in high amounts.

By limiting the intake of these foods, the risk of kidney stones reduces.

Can diet alone treat kidney stones?

For some people, dietary changes may be enough to prevent kidney stones from occurring.

In other cases, additional treatment may be necessary, including medication to break the stones up or surgery to remove the stones.

If stones become extremely painful, it is best to seek consultation with a doctor or nephrologist so they can recommend the best course of action.

7 DAY KIDNEY STONE DIET MEAL PLAN

The 7 day kidney stone diet meal plan to give you an idea of how you can structure your meals while focusing on preventing kidney stone formation. Remember to adjust portion sizes and specific foods based on your dietary needs, preferences, and any recommendations from a healthcare professional.

Day 1:

- Breakfast: Greek yogurt parfait with mixed berries and a sprinkle of granola.

- Lunch: Lentil and vegetable soup with a side salad.

- Snack: Carrot sticks with hummus.

- Dinner: Baked salmon with dill, roasted asparagus, and quinoa.

Day 2:

- Breakfast: Spinach and mushroom frittata with whole wheat toast.

- Lunch: Grilled chicken salad with mixed greens, cucumbers, and a light vina grette.

- Snack: Mixed nuts.

- Dinner: Brown rice stir-fry with tofu and assorted vegetables.

Day 3:

- Breakfast: Oatmeal topped with chopped nuts and fresh fruit.

- Lunch: Turkey and vegetable lettuce wraps with a side of sliced melon.

- Snack: Greek yogurt with a drizzle of honey.

- Dinner: Quinoa-stuffed bell peppers with a side salad.

Day 4:

- Breakfast: Whole grain cereal with almond milk and sliced banana.

- Lunch: Roasted vegetable medley served with a side of hummus and whole wheat pita.

- Snack: Apple slices with almond butter.

- Dinner: Chickpea and spinach curry served over brown rice.

Day 5:

- Breakfast: Scrambled eggs with sautéed spinach and whole grain toast.

- Lunch: Spinach and strawberry salad with walnuts and a balsamic vinaigrette.

- Snack: Cottage cheese and sliced peaches.

- Dinner: Lemon herb grilled chicken with quinoa and steamed broccoli.

Day 6:

- Breakfast: Berry and chia seed pudding.

- Lunch: Tuna salad with mixed greens and a lemon-tahini dressing.

- Snack: Fresh berries.

- Dinner: Baked eggplant Parmesan with a side of whole wheat spaghetti.

Day 7:

- Breakfast: Smoothie with kale, banana, almond milk, and a scoop of protein powder.

- Lunch: Veggie burger with sweet potato fries.

- Snack: Baby carrots with hummus.

- Dinner: Zucchini noodles with pesto and grilled shrimp skewers.

Remember to drink plenty of water throughout the day to maintain proper hydration. While following this meal plan, pay attention to portion sizes, and consult with a healthcare professional or registered dietitian if you have any specific dietary restrictions or medical concerns. They can help you personalize your meal plan to best suit your needs.

KIDNEY STONES DIET RECIPES

Baked Eggplant Parmesan:

Ingredients:

- 1 large eggplant, sliced into 1/4-inch rounds

- Salt, for drawing out moisture

- 1 cup all-purpose flour (for dredging)

- 2 large eggs, beaten

- 2 cups breadcrumbs (preferably Italian-style)

- Olive oil cooking spray

- 2 cups marinara sauce (store-bought or homemade)

- 2 cups shredded mozzarella cheese

- 1/2 cup grated Parmesan cheese

- Fresh basil leaves for garnish

Instructions:

1. Preheat the oven to 375°F (190°C).

2. Place the eggplant slices on a baking sheet and sprinkle salt on both sides. Let them sit for about 20-30 minutes to draw out excess moisture.

Afterward, pat the eggplant slices dry with paper towels.

3. Set up a dredging station: Place the flour in one shallow dish, beaten eggs in another dish, and breadcrumbs in a th rd dish.

4. Dredge each eggplant slice in the flour, then dip it into the beaten eggs, and coat it with breadcrumbs. Press the breadcrumbs gertly onto the eggplant to ensure even coating.

5. Place the coated eggplant slices on a baking sheet lined with parchment paper.

6. Lightly spray the coated eggplant slices with olive oil cooking spray.

7. Bake the eggplant slices in the preheated oven for about 20-25 minutes, flipping them halfway through, until they are golden and crispy.

8. In a baking dish, spread a thin layer of marinara sauce on the bottom.

9. Place a layer of baked eggplant slices on top of the sauce.

10. Spoon a little more marinara sauce over the eggplant slices.

11. Sprinkle shredded mozzarella cheese over the sauce.

12. Repeat the layers: eggplant, sauce, and cheese until you've used all the ingredients.

13. Finish with a layer of grated Parmesan cheese on top.

14. Bake the eggplant Parmesan in the oven for about 20-25 minutes, or until the cheese is melted and bubbly.

15. Let the dish cool slightly before serving.

16. Garnish with fresh basil leaves before serving.

17. Serve the baked eggplant Parmesan as a flavorful and satisfying main dish.

This baked eggplant Parmesan provides a tasty alternative to the traditional fried version while still offering the same delicious flavors. It's a suitable option for a kidney stone diet, especially when enjoyed in moderation due to the cheese content.

Berry and Chia Seed Pudding

Here's a simple recipe for Berry and Chia Seed Pudding:

Ingredients:

- 1/4 cup chia seeds

- 1 cup unsweetened almond milk (or any milk of your choice)

- 1 teaspoon honey or maple syrup (adjust to taste)

- 1/2 teaspoon vanilla extract

- Mixed berries (such as strawberries, blueberries, raspberries) for topping

- Optional: sliced almonds or chopped nuts for extra crunch

Instructions:

1. In a bowl, combine chia seeds, almond milk, honey or maple syrup, and vanilla extract. Mix well to ensure the chia seeds are evenly distributed.

2. Cover the bowl and place it in the refrigerator for at least 2-3 hours, or preferably overnight. This allows the chia seeds to absorb the liquid and create a pudding-like consistency.

3. After the chia seeds have absorbed the liquid and the mixture has thickened, give it a good stir to break up any clumps.

4. Serve the chia seed pudding in individual bowls or glasses. Top with a generous amount of mixed berries and optional sliced almonds or chopped nuts.

5. Enjoy the pudding as a healthy and satisfying breakfast, snack, or dessert!

Feel free to customize the recipe by adding other toppings like shredded coconut, granola, or a drizzle of nut butter. Adjust the sweetness and flavors to your preference. This recipe provides a nutritious and tasty option for those following a kidney stone diet.

Quinoa and Black Bean Bowl

Here's a recipe for a Quinoa and Black Bean Bowl:

Ingredients:

- 1 cup quinoa, rinsed and drained

- 2 cups water or vegetable broth

- 1 can (15 oz) black beans, drained and rinsed

- 1 cup corn kernels (fresh, frozen, or canned)

- 1 red bell pepper, diced

- 1 avocado, diced

- 1/4 cup chopped fresh cilantro

- Juice of 1 lime

- Salt and pepper, to taste

- Optional toppings: diced tomatoes, shredded cheese, Greek yogurt, salsa

Instructions:

1. In a medium saucepan, bring the water or vegetable broth to a boil. Add the quinoa and reduce the heat to low. Cover and let the quinoa simmer for about 15-20 minutes, or until the liquid is absorbed and the quinoa is cooked. Fluff the quinoa with a fork.

2. In a large mixing bowl, combine the cooked quinoa, black beans, corn kernels, diced red bell pepper, diced avocado, and chopped cilantro.

3. Squeeze the lime juice over the quinoa mixture and toss everything together.

4. Season the quinoa and black bean mixture with salt and pepper to taste. Adjust the seasoning as needed.

5. Divide the quinoa and black bean mixture into serving bowls.

6. If desired, top the bowls with additional toppings such as diced tomatoes, shredded cheese, a dollop of Greek yogurt, or salsa.

7. Serve the quinoa and black bean bowl as a nutritious and satisfying meal.

This quinoa and black bean bowl is an excellent option for a kidney stone diet, providing a good source of protein, fiber, and various vitamins and minerals. It's a versatile dish that can be customized with your favorite vegetables and toppings. Enjoy!

Orange and Almond Salad

Here's a recipe for Orange and Almond Salad with Mixed Greens:

Ingredients:

-   4 cups mixed salad greens (such as lettuce, spinach, arugula)

-   2 large oranges, peeled and segmented

-   1/4 cup sliced almonds

- 1/4 cup crumbled feta cheese (optional)

- 2 tablespoons extra-virgin olive oil

- 1 tablespoon balsamic vinegar

- 1 teaspoon honey

- Salt and pepper to taste

Instructions:

1. In a large salad bowl, combine the mixed salad greens. You can use a variety of greens for a colorful and flavorful salad.

2. Add the orange segments to the greens. Gently toss the salad to combine the greens and oranges.

3. In a small dry skillet, toast the sliced almonds over medium heat until they are lightly golden and fragrant. Keep a close eye on them to prevent burning. Remove from heat and set aside.

4. If using, sprinkle the crumbled feta cheese over the salad.

5. In a small bowl, whisk together the extra-virgin olive oil, balsamic vinegar, honey, salt, and pepper. This will be the dressing for the salad.

6. Drizzle the dressing over the salad and toss gently to coat the greens, oranges, and any additional toppings.

7. Sprinkle the toasted sliced almonds on top of the salad for added crunch and nutty flavor.

8. Serve the orange and almond salad immediately as a refreshing and nutritious appetizer or side dish.

Feel free to adjust the quantities of ingredients based on your preferences. This salad provides a great combination of flavors and textures, making it a delicious addition to a kidney stone diet. Enjoy!

Cottage Cheese

Here's a simple recipe for a Cottage Cheese and Fruit Bowl:

Ingredients:

- 1 cup low-fat cottage cheese

- 1 cup mixed fresh fruits (such as berries, sliced banana, diced mango, or kiwi)

- 1 tablespoon honey or maple syrup (optional)

- 2 tablespoons chopped nuts (such as almonds, walnuts, or pistachios)

-    Fresh mint leaves for garnish (optional)

Instructions:

1. In a bowl, scoop the low-fat cottage cheese as the base.

2. Arrange the mixed fresh fruits on top of the cottage cheese.

3. If desired, drizzle honey or maple syrup over the fruit for a touch of sweetness.

4. Sprinkle the chopped nuts over the fruit and cottage cheese mixture.

5. Garnish with fresh mint leaves for added freshness and color.

6. Serve the cottage cheese and fruit bowl as a wholesome and balanced breakfast, snack, or light meal.

This cottage cheese and fruit bowl is a great choice for a kidney stone diet, as it provides protein, fiber, vitamins, and minerals from the cottage cheese and fresh fruits. It's a refreshing and nutritious option that's quick and easy to prepare. Enjoy!

Cauliflower Mash with Roasted Garlic:

Ingredients:

- 1 head cauliflower, cut into florets

- 1 bulb of garlic

- 2 tablespoons olive oil

- Salt and pepper, to taste

- 1/4 cup unsweetened almond milk (or milk of your choice)

- 2 tablespoons unsalted butter or olive oil

- Fresh chopped parsley or chives for garnish (optional)

Instructions:

1. Preheat the oven to 400°F (200°C).

2. Cut off the top of the garlic bulb to expose the cloves. Drizzle a bit of olive oil over the exposed cloves, then wrap the bulb in aluminum foil. Place the wrapped garlic bulb on a baking sheet and roast in the preheated oven for about 30-35 minutes, until the cloves are soft and golden.

3. While the garlic is roasting, steam or boil the cauliflower florets until they are tender. This usually takes about 10-15 minutes.

4. Drain the cooked cauliflower and transfer it to a food processor or blender.

5. Squeeze the roasted garlic cloves out of the bulb and add them to the blender or food processor with the cauliflower.

6. Add the unsweetened almond milk, butter or olive oil, salt, and pepper to the blender or food processor.

7. Blend or process the mixture until smooth and creamy, similar to the texture of mashed potatoes. You might need to stop and scrape down the sides a few times to ensure everything is well combined.

8. Taste the cauliflower mash and adjust the seasoning if needed.

9. Transfer the cauliflower mash to a serving bowl and garnish with chopped parsley or chives, if desired.

10. Serve the cauliflower mash as a delicious and lower-carb alternative to traditional mashed potatoes.

This cauliflower mash is a great side dish for a kidney stone diet, as it provides a creamy texture without the excess potassium found in regular potatoes. Enjoy!

Turkey and Vegetable Stir-Fry:

Ingredients:

- 1 pound ground turkey

- 2 tablespoons soy sauce (or tamari for gluten-free)

- 1 tablespoon oyster sauce (optional)

- 1 tablespoon hoisin sauce

- 1 tablespoon sesame oil

- 1 tablespoon olive oil

- 2 cloves garlic, minced

- 1 teaspoon fresh ginger, minced

- 1 cup sliced bell peppers (a mix of colors)

- 1 cup broccoli florets

- 1 cup snap peas or snow peas, trimmed

- 1 carrot, julienned or thinly sliced

- 1/4 cup chopped green onions (scallions)

- Salt and pepper, to taste

- Sesame seeds for garnish (optional)

- Cooked brown rice or quinoa, for serving

Instructions:

1. In a small bowl, whisk together the soy sauce, oyster sauce (if using), hoisin sauce, and sesame oil. Set aside.

2. In a large skillet or wok, heat the olive oil over medium-high heat.

3. Add the minced garlic and fresh ginger to the skillet. Sauté for about 1 minute until fragrant.

4. Add the ground turkey to the skillet. Cook, breaking it up with a spatula, until it's browned and cooked through.

5. Pour the sauce mixture over the cooked turkey and stir to coat the meat evenly.

6. Add the sliced bell peppers, broccoli florets, snap peas or snow peas, and julienned carrot to the skillet. Stir-fry for about 3-4 minutes until the vegetables are tender-crisp.

7. Add chopped green onions to the skillet and stir to combine.

8. Taste the stir-fry and adjust the seasoning with salt and pepper if needed.

9. Remove the skillet from the heat.

10. Serve the turkey and vegetable stir-fry over cooked brown rice or quinoa.

11. If desired, sprinkle sesame seeds over the top for added texture and flavor.

12. Enjoy the turkey and vegetable stir-fry as a delicious and balanced meal.

This turkey and vegetable stir-fry is a nutritious option for a kidney stone diet, as it offers lean protein and a variety of colorful vegetables. It's a quick and flavorful dish that's perfect for busy weeknight dinners.

Broccoli and White Bean Soup

Here's a recipe for Broccoli and White Bean Soup:

Ingredients:

- 2 cups broccoli florets

- 1 can (15 oz) white beans (such as cannellini beans), drained and rinsed

- 1 small onion, chopped

- 2 cloves garlic, minced

- 4 cups vegetable broth

- 1 teaspoon dried thyme

- 1/2 teaspoon dried oregano

- Salt and pepper, to taste

- 2 tablespoons olive oil

- Optional toppings: grated Parmesan cheese, chopped fresh parsley

Instructions:

1. In a large pot, heat the olive oil over medium heat. Add the chopped onion and cook until it becomes translucent, about 3-4 minutes.

2. Add the minced garlic and cook for an additional 1 minute until fragrant.

3. Add the broccoli florets to the pot and sauté for about 5 minutes, until they start to soften.

4. Pour in the vegetable broth and bring the mixture to a simmer. Let it cook for about 10-15 minutes, until the broccoli is tender.

5. Add the drained and rinsed white beans to the pot.

6. Use an immersion blender to puree the soup until smooth. Alternatively, you can carefully transfer the soup in batches to a regular blender and

blend until smooth. Just be cautious when blending hot liquids.

7. Return the blended soup to the pot if needed. Stir in the dried thyme, dried oregano, salt, and pepper. Adjust the seasonings to your taste.

8. Let the soup simmer for another 5-10 minutes to allow the flavors to meld together.

9. Once the soup is heated through and well seasoned, ladle it into serving bowls.

10. If desired, sprinkle grated Parmesan cheese and chopped fresh parsley on top before serving.

11. Enjoy the creamy and nutritious broccoli and white bean soup as a comforting meal.

This soup is rich in fiber, protein, and vitamins, making it a great choice for a kidney stone diet. It's also a satisfying and flavorful option for anyone looking for a hearty soup.

Steamed Asparagus

Here's a simple recipe for Steamed Asparagus with Lemon Zest:

Ingredients:

-   1 bunch of fresh asparagus

-   1 lemon

-   Olive oil

-   Salt and pepper, to taste

Instructions:

1. Wash the asparagus thoroughly and trim the tough ends by snapping them off where they naturally break.

2. Prepare a pot or steamer with water for steaming the asparagus.

3. Place the asparagus in the steamer basket and steam them for about 3-5 minutes, or until they are tender but still slightly crisp.

4. While the asparagus is steaming, zest the lemon using a fine grater to get the outer yellow peel. Be sure to avoid grating the bitter white pith underneath.

5. Once the asparagus is done steaming, remove them from the steamer basket and place them on a serving platter.

6. Drizzle a little olive oil over the steamed asparagus.

7. Sprinkle the lemon zest over the asparagus.

8. Season the asparagus with a pinch of salt and freshly ground black pepper.

9. Gently toss the asparagus to coat them with the olive oil and lemon zest.

10. Serve the steamed asparagus with lemon zest as a light and flavorful side dish.

This steamed asparagus with lemon zest is a great choice for a kidney stone diet, as asparagus is low in oxalates and offers various vitamins and minerals. The addition of lemon zest adds a burst of citrusy flavor that complements the asparagus perfectly. Enjoy!

Cucumber and Avocado Sushi Rolls

Here's a recipe for Cucumber and Avocado Sushi Rolls:

Ingredients:

- 2 cups sushi rice, cooked and seasoned (seasoned with rice vinegar, sugar, and salt)

- Nori (seaweed) sheets

- 1 avocado, thinly sliced

- 1 cucumber, julienned

- Soy sauce, for dipping

- Wasabi and pickled ginger, for serving (optional)

Instructions:

1. Lay a bamboo sushi rolling mat on a clean surface and place a sheet of plastic wrap on top of it. This will prevent the rice from sticking to the mat.

2. Place a sheet of nori, shiny side down, on the plastic wrap. Wet your fingers with water to prevent sticking, and evenly spread a layer of sushi rice over the nori, leaving about 1/2 inch of nori exposed at the top edge.

3. Lay thin slices of avocado and julienned cucumber horizontally along the center of the rice.

4. Begin rolling the sushi by using the bamboo mat to lift and fold the bottom edge of the nori over the filling. Use gentle pressure to start rolling, making sure the filling is enclosed.

5. Continue rolling, using the bamboo mat to help shape the roll and keep it tight. Roll until you reach the exposed edge of the nori.

6. Wet the exposed nori edge with a little water to seal the roll. Continue rolling until the roll is completely sealed.

7. Use a sharp knife to slice the sushi roll into bite-sized pieces. Dip the knife in water between cuts to prevent sticking.

8. Arrange the sliced sushi rolls on a plate.

9. Serve the cucumber and avocado sushi rolls with soy sauce for dipping. If you like, you can also offer wasabi and pickled ginger on the side.

10. Enjoy your homemade sushi rolls as a delicious and healthy meal or snack!

These sushi rolls are a wonderful option for a kidney stone diet, as they contain fresh vegetables, healthy fats, and nutrient-rich ingredients. Plus, making your own sushi at home allows you to customize the ingredients to your liking.

Oatmeal with Chopped Nuts and Fresh Fruit

Here's a simple recipe for Oatmeal with Chopped Nuts and Fresh Fruit:

Ingredients:

-   1 cup rolled oats

- 2 cups water or milk (dairy or plant-based)

- Pinch of salt

- Chopped nuts (such as almonds, walnuts, or pecans)

- Fresh fruit (such as berries, sliced banana, diced apple, or pear)

- Honey or maple syrup, for sweetness (optional)

Instructions:

1. In a saucepan, bring the water or milk and a pinch of salt to a boil.

2. Stir in the rolled oats and reduce the heat to medium-low.

3. Cook the oats, stirring occasionally, for about 5-7 minutes, or until they are creamy and have absorbed most of the liquid.

4. Once the oats are cooked to your desired consistency, remove the saucepan from the heat.

5. Spoon the cooked oatmeal into serving bowls.

6. Top the oatmeal with chopped nuts for added crunch and a dose of healthy fats.

7. Add your choice of fresh fruit over the oatmeal. Berries, sliced banana, diced apple, or pear work well.

8. If desired, drizzle a little honey or maple syrup over the oatmeal for sweetness.

9. Give the oatmeal a gentle stir to mix in the toppings.

10. Serve the oatmeal with chopped nuts and fresh fruit as a wholesome and comforting breakfast.

This oatmeal with chopped nuts and fresh fruit is a nutritious and filling option for a kidney stone diet, providing fiber, vitamins, and minerals. It's a versatile dish that can be customized with your favorite nuts and fruits. Enjoy!

Baked Chicken with Herbed Quinoa

Here's a recipe for Baked Chicken with Herbed Quinoa:

Ingredients for Baked Chicken:

-   2 boneless, skinless chicken breasts

-   2 tablespoons olive oil

-   1 teaspoon dried thyme

-     1 teaspoon dried rosemary

-     Salt and pepper, to taste

Ingredients for Herbed Quinoa:

-     1 cup quinoa, rinsed and drained

-     2 cups chicken or vegetable broth

-     1 teaspoon dried oregano

-     1 teaspoon dried basil

-     Salt and pepper, to taste

Instructions:

1.   Preheat the oven to 375°F (190°C).

2.   In a small bowl, mix together the olive oil, dried thyme, dried rosemary, salt, and pepper. Brush the mixture over both sides of the chicken breasts.

3.   Heat an oven-safe skillet over medium-high heat. Once hot, add the chicken breasts and cook for about 2-3 minutes on each side to sear and brown the outside.

4.   Transfer the skillet to the preheated oven and bake the chicken for about 15-20 minutes, or until the internal temperature reaches 165°F (74°C) and the chicken is cooked through.

5.   While the chicken is baking, prepare the herbed quinoa. In a medium saucepan, combine the rinsed quinoa, chicken or vegetable broth, dried oregano, dried basil, salt, and pepper.

6.   Bring the mixture to a boil, then reduce the heat to low, cover, and let it simmer for about 15 minutes, or until the quinoa is cooked and the liquid is absorbed.

7.   Fluff the cooked quinoa with a fork and adjust the seasoning if needed.

8.   Once the chicken is done baking, remove it from the oven and let it rest for a few minutes before slicing.

9.   To serve, spoon a portion of the herbed quinoa onto each plate and top with slices of baked chicken.

10. Enjoy your flavorful and nutritious baked chicken with herbed quinoa!

This dish provides a balanced combination of protein, whole grains, and herbs, making it a satisfying and wholesome choice for a kidney stone diet. Feel free to add steamed vegetables or a side salad to complete the meal.

Cucumber and Tomato Salad

Here's a recipe for a refreshing Cucumber and Tomato Salad with Basil:

Ingredients:

- 2 cups diced cucumbers (English cucumber works well)

- 2 cups diced tomatoes (use a mix of cherry tomatoes or vine-ripened tomatoes)

- 1/4 cup thinly sliced red onion

- 1/4 cup chopped fresh basil leaves

- 2 tablespoons extra-virgin olive oil

- 1 tablespoon balsamic vinegar

- Salt and pepper, to taste

Instructions:

1. In a large bowl, combine the diced cucumbers, diced tomatoes, thinly sliced red onion, and chopped fresh basil.

2. In a small bowl, whisk together the extra-virgin olive oil and balsamic vinegar to make the dressing.

3. Drizzle the dressing over the cucumber and
    tomato mixture.

4. Gently toss the salad to coat the ingredients
    with the dressing.

5. Season the salad with salt and pepper to taste.

6. Allow the flavors to meld for about 10-15
    minutes before serving, if possible.

7. Serve the cucumber and tomato salad with basil
    as a light and refreshing side dish.

This cucumber and tomato salad with basil is an
excellent option for a kidney stone diet, as it's hydrating,
low in oxalates, and provides a variety of vitamins and
minerals. The addition of fresh basil adds a burst of
herbal flavor that complements the vegetables
beautifully. Enjoy!

Greek Yogurt Smoothie

Here's a recipe for a refreshing Greek Yogurt Smoothie
with Mango:

Ingredients:

-   1 cup Greek yogurt (plain or vanilla)

-   1 ripe mango, peeled, pitted, and chopped

-     1/2 cup unsweetened almond milk (or any milk of your choice)

-     1 tablespoon honey or maple syrup (adjust to taste)

-     1/2 teaspoon vanilla extract

-     Ice cubes (optional)

-     Fresh mint leaves for garnish (optional)

Instructions:

1. In a blender, combine the Greek yogurt, chopped mango, almond milk, honey or maple syrup, and vanilla extract.

2. If desired, add a handful of ice cubes to the blender for a colder and thicker smoothie.

3. Blend all the ingredients until smooth and creamy. If the consistency is too thick, you can add a little more almond milk to reach your desired thickness.

4. Taste the smoothie and adjust the sweetness by adding more honey or maple syrup if needed.

5. Pour the smoothie into glasses and garnish with fresh mint leaves, if desired.

6. Serve the Greek yogurt smoothie with mango immediately for a delicious and nutritious drink.

This smoothie is a great source of protein from the Greek yogurt and vitamins from the mango, making it a suitable option for a kidney stone diet. It's a wonderful way to enjoy the natural sweetness of mango while staying hydrated and nourished.

Chickpea and Spinach Curry

Here's a recipe for Chickpea and Spinach Curry:

Ingredients:

- 1 tablespoon olive oil

- 1 onion, finely chopped

- 2 cloves garlic, minced

- 1 teaspoon fresh ginger, minced

- 1 tablespoon curry powder

- 1 teaspoon ground cumin

- 1 teaspoon ground coriander

- 1/2 teaspoon turmeric

- 1/4 teaspoon cayenne pepper (adjust to taste)

- 1 can (15 oz) chickpeas, drained and rinsed

- 1 can (14 oz) diced tomatoes

- 1 can (14 oz) coconut milk

- 4 cups fresh spinach leaves

- Salt and pepper, to taste

- Juice of 1 lemon

- Fresh cilantro leaves for garnish

- Cooked rice or naan bread, for serving

Instructions:

1. In a large skillet or pot, heat the olive oil over medium heat.

2. Add the chopped onion and sauté for about 2-3 minutes, until it becomes translucent.

3. Stir in the minced garlic and minced ginger, and cook for another 1-2 minutes until fragrant.

4. Add the curry powder, ground cumin, ground coriander, turmeric, and cayenne pepper to the skillet. Stir and cook the spices for about 1 minute to toast them.

5. Pour in the diced tomatoes (with their juices) and coconut milk. Stir to combine and bring the mixture to a simmer.

6. Add the drained and rinsed chickpeas to the skillet. Stir and let the curry simmer for about 10-15 minutes to allow the flavors to meld.

7. Gently fold in the fresh spinach leaves and let them wilt in the curry.

8. Season the curry with salt and pepper to taste.

9. Squeeze the lemon juice over the curry and stir to incorporate.

10. Once the spinach is wilted and the chickpeas are heated through, remove the skillet from the heat.

11. Serve the chickpea and spinach curry over cooked rice or with naan bread.

12. Garnish with fresh cilantro leaves for added flavor and freshness.

13. Enjoy the chickpea and spinach curry as a flavorful and nutritious main dish.

This chickpea and spinach curry is a fantastic choice for a kidney stone diet, as it's rich in fiber, plant-based protein, and a variety of spices that add both flavor and potential health benefits. Pair it with whole grains or bread for a well-rounded meal.

Here's a simple recipe for Roasted Portobello Mushrooms with Herbs:

Ingredients:

- 4 large Portobello mushrooms

- 3 tablespoons olive oil

- 2 cloves garlic, minced

- 1 tablespoon fresh thyme leaves (or 1 teaspoon dried thyme)

- 1 tablespoon fresh rosemary leaves (or 1 teaspoon dried rosemary)

- Salt and pepper, to taste

- Grated Parmesan cheese for garnish (optional)

- Chopped fresh parsley for garnish (optional)

Instructions:

1. Preheat the oven to 375°F (190°C).

2. Clean the Portobello mushrooms by gently wiping them with a damp cloth or paper towel. Remove the stems and scrape out the gills using a spoon.

3. In a small bowl, mix together the olive oil, minced garlic, fresh thyme, fresh rosemary, salt, and pepper.

4. Brush the olive oil and herb mixture over both sides of the Portobello mushrooms, making sure to coat them evenly.

5. Place the mushrooms on a baking sheet, gill-side up.

6. Roast the mushrooms in the preheated oven for about 15-20 minutes, or until they are tender and cooked through. The cooking time may vary depending on the size of the mushrooms.

7. Once the mushrooms are done roasting, remove them from the oven and transfer them to a serving plate.

8. If desired, sprinkle grated Parmesan cheese over the mushrooms while they are still warm.

9. Garnish the roasted Portobello mushrooms with chopped fresh parsley for added flavor and color.

10. Serve the mushrooms as a tasty appetizer or side dish.

These roasted Portobello mushrooms are low in calories and provide a rich and savory flavor. They can be a great addition to a kidney stone diet, offering a delicious and nutritious alternative to meat-based dishes. Enjoy!

Grilled Shrimp Skewers

Here's a recipe for Grilled Shrimp Skewers with Pineapple:

Ingredients:

- 1 pound large shrimp, peeled and deveined

- 1 cup pineapple chunks

- 2 tablespoons olive oil

- 2 cloves garlic, minced

- 1 teaspoon paprika

- 1/2 teaspoon ground cumin

- Salt and pepper, to taste

- Wooden skewers, soaked in water

- Fresh cilantro leaves for garnish

- Lime wedges for serving

1. In a bowl, whisk together the olive oil, minced garlic, paprika, ground cumin, salt, and pepper to create the marinade.

2. Add the peeled and deveined shrimp to the marinade and toss to coat them evenly. Let them marinate for about 15-20 minutes.

3. Preheat the grill to medium-high heat.

4. Thread the marinated shrimp onto the soaked wooden skewers, alternating with pineapple chunks.

5. Place the shrimp skewers on the preheated grill and cook for about 2-3 minutes on each side, or until the shrimp are pink and opaque.

6. While grilling, you can brush any remaining marinade onto the shrimp for extra flavor.

7. Once the shrimp are cooked through, remove them from the grill.

8. Garnish the grilled shrimp skewers with fresh cilantro leaves.

9. Serve the skewers with lime wedges on the side for a burst of citrusy freshness.

10. Enjoy the grilled shrimp skewers with pineapple as a tasty and protein-rich main dish.

These grilled shrimp skewers with pineapple are a delicious option for a kidney stone diet, offering lean protein from the shrimp and the natural sweetness of the pineapple. They make for a delightful summer meal that's both flavorful and satisfying.

Vegetable and Lentil Stew

Here's a recipe for Vegetable and Lentil Stew:

Ingredients:

- 1 cup dried green or brown lentils, rinsed and drained

- 1 tablespoon olive oil

- 1 onion, chopped

- 2 carrots, peeled and chopped

- 2 celery stalks, chopped

- 2 cloves garlic, minced

- 1 teaspoon ground cumin

- 1 teaspoon ground coriander

- 1/2 teaspoon ground turmeric

- 1/2 teaspoon smoked paprika (optional)

- 1 can (14 oz) diced tomatoes

- 4 cups vegetable broth

- 2 cups chopped mixed vegetables (such as bell peppers, zucchini, and spinach)

- Salt and pepper, to taste

- Fresh chopped parsley for garnish

Instructions:

1. In a large pot, heat the olive oil over medium heat. Add the chopped onion, carrots, and celery. Sauté for about 5-7 minutes, until the vegetables start to soften.

2. Add the minced garlic, ground cumin, ground coriander, ground turmeric, and smoked paprika (if using). Cook for another 1-2 minutes until the spices are fragrant.

3. Add the rinsed lentils, diced tomatoes (with their juices), and vegetable broth to the pot. Stir to combine.

4. Bring the mixture to a simmer and let it cook for about 20-25 minutes, until the lentils are tender.

5. Add the chopped mixed vegetables to the stew and cook for an additional 10-15 minutes, or until the vegetables are cooked to your liking.

6. Season the stew with salt and pepper to taste. Adjust the seasoning as needed.

7. Once the lentils and vegetables are cooked and the flavors have melded together, remove the pot from the heat.

8. Ladle the vegetable and lentil stew into serving bowls and garnish with fresh chopped parsley.

9. Enjoy the hearty and flavorful vegetable and lentil stew as a nourishing meal.

This stew is packed with fiber, protein, and a variety of vegetables, making it a great option for a kidney stone diet. It's a comforting and satisfying dish that's perfect for colder weather or anytime you're craving a wholesome meal.

Mixed Berry and Spinach Smoothie

Here's a recipe for a Mixed Berry and Spinach Smoothie:

Ingredients:

- 1 cup mixed berries (such as strawberries, blueberries, raspberries)

- 1 cup fresh spinach leaves

- 1 ripe banana

- 1/2 cup plain Greek yogurt

- 1/2 cup unsweetened almond milk (or any milk of your choice)

- 1 tablespoon chia seeds (optional)

- Honey or maple syrup, to taste (optional)

- Ice cubes

Instructions:

1. In a blender, combine the mixed berries, fresh spinach leaves, ripe banana, plain Greek yogurt, unsweetened almond milk, and chia seeds (if using).

2. If you prefer a sweeter smoothie, add honey or maple syrup to taste.

3. Add a handful of ice cubes to the blender to make the smoothie cold and refreshing.

4. Blend on high speed until all the ingredients are well combined and the smoothie is creamy and smooth.

5. Taste the smoothie and adjust the sweetness if
    needed by adding more honey or maple syrup.

6. Pour the mixed berry and spinach smoothie into
    glasses.

7. If desired, garnish with a few additional berries or
    a sprinkle of chia seeds.

8. Serve the smoothie immediately as a nutritious
    and delicious breakfast or snack.

This mixed berry and spinach smoothie is a great choice
for a kidney stone diet, as it combines the vitamins and
antioxidants from the berries with the nutrients from
spinach, without being high in oxalates. The Greek
yogurt adds protein and creaminess, while the chia
seeds provide healthy omega-3 fatty acids and fiber.
Enjoy!

Sautéed Shrimp with Garlic

Here's a recipe for Sautéed Shrimp with Garlic and
Lemon:

Ingredients:

-   1 pound large shrimp, peeled and deveined

-   2 tablespoons olive oil

- 4 cloves garlic, minced

- Zest of 1 lemon

- Juice of 1 lemon

- Salt and pepper, to taste

- Fresh chopped parsley for garnish

- Optional: red pepper flakes for a bit of heat

Instructions:

1. In a bowl, combine the peeled and deveined shrimp with the minced garlic, lemon zest, and a pinch of salt and pepper. Toss to coat the shrimp with the flavors.

2. Heat the olive oil in a large skillet over medium-high heat.

3. Add the seasoned shrimp to the skillet in a single layer. Cook for about 2-3 minutes on each side, until the shrimp turn pink and opaque. Be careful not to overcook them, as shrimp cook quickly.

4. Squeeze the juice of one lemon over the cooked shrimp in the skillet. If you like a bit of heat, you can also add a pinch of red pepper flakes at this point.

5. Give everything a quick toss to ensure the shrimp are evenly coated with the lemon juice and garlic.

6.   Remove the skillet from the heat.

7.   Serve the sautéed shrimp with garlic and lemon in a serving dish, garnished with fresh chopped parsley.

8.   Enjoy the delicious and flavorful sautéed shrimp as a protein-rich dish.

This shrimp dish is a wonderful option for a kidney stone diet, as it's low in saturated fat and provides lean protein. The combination of garlic and lemon adds a burst of flavor to the shrimp. You can pair it with a side of steamed vegetables or a light salad for a well-rounded meal.

Zucchini Noodles with Pesto

Here's a recipe for Zucchini Noodles with Pesto:

Ingredients:

For the Zucchini Noodles:

- 2-3 medium zucchinis

- Salt

For the Pesto:

- 2 cups fresh basil leaves

- 1/2 cup grated Parmesan cheese

- 1/2 cup pine nuts or walnuts

- 2 cloves garlic, peeled

- 1/2 cup extra-virgin olive oil

- Salt and pepper, to taste

- Juice of 1 lemon (optional)

Instructions:

For the Zucchini Noodles:

1. Wash and trim the ends of the zucchinis.

2. Using a spiralizer or a vegetable peeler, create thin zucchini noodles.

3. Place the zucchini noodles in a colander, sprinkle them with a little salt, and let them sit for about 10-15 minutes. This helps draw out excess moisture.

4. After the resting time, gently squeeze the zucchini noodles to remove any excess water.

For the Pesto:

1. In a food processor, combine the fresh basil leaves, grated Parmesan cheese, pine nuts or walnuts, and peeled garlic cloves.

2. Pulse until the ingredients are finely chopped and blended.

3. With the food processor running, gradually drizzle in the extra-virgin olive oil until the pesto reaches a smooth and creamy consistency.

4. Season the pesto with salt and pepper to taste. If desired, add the juice of 1 lemon for a tangy kick.

To Assemble:

1. In a large bowl, toss the zucchini noodles with the desired amount of pesto, coating them evenly.

2. Serve the zucchini noodles with pesto as a light and flavorful dish.

3. You can enjoy the dish as is or top it with additional grated Parmesan cheese and chopped fresh basil.

This zucchini noodles with pesto dish is a wonderful option for a kidney stone diet, as it offers a low-carb alternative to traditional pasta and a fresh, herbaceous pesto sauce. It's a great way to enjoy the flavors of summer in a healthy and satisfying manner.

Apple and Walnut Quinoa Bowl

Here's a recipe for an Apple and Walnut Quinoa Bowl:

- 1 cup quinoa, rinsed and drained

- 2 cups water or vegetable broth

- 1 large apple, cored and diced

- 1/2 cup chopped walnuts

- 1/4 cup dried cranberries or raisins

- 1 teaspoon cinnamon

- 1 tablespoon honey or maple syrup

- Greek yogurt or almond milk for serving (optional)

Instructions:

1. In a medium saucepan, bring the water or vegetable broth to a boil. Add the quinoa and reduce the heat to low. Cover and let the quinoa simmer for about 15-20 minutes, or until the liquid is absorbed and the quinoa is cooked. Fluff the quinoa with a fork.

2. In a large bowl, combine the cooked quinoa, diced apple, chopped walnuts, dried cranberries or raisins, and cinnamon.

3. Drizzle the honey or maple syrup over the quinoa mixture and give it a good toss to coat everything evenly.

4. Taste and adjust the sweetness or cinnamon level if desired.

5. Serve the apple and walnut quinoa mixture in bowls.

6. If desired, you can top each bowl with a dollop of Greek yogurt or a splash of almond milk.

7. Enjoy the wholesome and satisfying apple and walnut quinoa bowl as a nourishing breakfast or snack.

This quinoa bowl provides a good balance of whole grains, fruits, and healthy fats, making it a suitable choice for a kidney stone diet. It's a delightful way to incorporate seasonal fruits and nuts into your meals.

Sweet Potato and Black Bean Tacos

Here's a recipe for Sweet Potato and Black Bean Tacos:

Ingredients:

For the Sweet Potato Filling:

- 2 medium sweet potatoes, peeled and diced

- 2 tablespoons olive oil

- 1 teaspoon ground cumin

- 1/2 teaspoon chili powder

- Salt and pepper, to taste

For the Black Bean Filling:

- 1 can (15 oz) black beans, drained and rinsed

- 1 teaspoon ground cumin

- 1/2 teaspoon chili powder

- Salt and pepper, to taste

For Assembling the Tacos:

- Corn or whole wheat tortillas

- Sliced avocado

- Chopped fresh cilantro

- Salsa or pico de gallo

- Lime wedges

Instructions:

For the Sweet Potato Filling:

1. Preheat the oven to 400°F (200°C).

2. In a bowl, toss the diced sweet potatoes with olive oil, ground cumin, chili powder, salt, and pepper.

3. Spread the seasoned sweet potatoes on a baking sheet in a single layer.

4. Roast the sweet potatoes in the preheated oven for about 20-25 minutes, or until they are tender and slightly crispy on the edges.

For the Black Bean Filling:

1. In a saucepan, combine the drained and rinsed black beans, ground cumin, chili powder, salt, and pepper.

2. Heat the bean mixture over medium heat until it's warmed through.

To Assemble the Tacos:

1. Warm the tortillas according to the package instructions.

2. Spoon some of the roasted sweet potato filling onto each tortilla.

3. Top the sweet potatoes with a scoop of the black bean filling.

4. Add sliced avocado, chopped fresh cilantro, and a spoonful of salsa or pico de gallo on top.

5. Squeeze fresh lime juice over the fillings.

6. Fold the tortillas and enjoy the sweet potato and black bean tacos.

These sweet potato and black bean tacos are a fantastic option for a kidney stone diet, offering a balance of flavors, fiber, and plant-based protein. Customize the toppings to your liking and savor a delicious and nutritious meal.

Veggie Burger with Sweet Potato Fries

Here's a recipe for a Veggie Burger with Sweet Potato Fries:

Ingredients for Veggie Burger:

- 1 can (15 oz) black beans, drained and rinsed

- 1 cup cooked quinoa

- 1/2 cup finely chopped onion

- 1/2 cup grated carrot

- 1/4 cup chopped bell pepper (any color)

- 2 cloves garlic, minced

- 1 teaspoon ground cumin

- 1 teaspoon paprika

- Salt and pepper, to taste

- 1/4 cup breadcrumbs (adjust as needed)

- Olive oil for cooking

- 2 large sweet potatoes, peeled and cut into fries

- 2 tablespoons olive oil

- 1 teaspoon paprika

- Salt and pepper, to taste

For assembling:

- Whole grain burger buns

- Lettuce leaves

- Sliced tomatoes

- Condiments of your choice (mayonnaise, ketchup, mustard)

Instructions:

For Veggie Burger:

1. In a large mixing bowl, mash the black beans using a fork or potato masher until mostly smooth, leaving some texture.

2. Add the cooked quinoa, chopped onion, grated carrot, chopped bel pepper, minced garlic, ground cumin, paprika, salt. and pepper to the mashed beans. Mix well to combine.

3. Stir in the breadcrumbs gradually until the mixture holds together well and is not too sticky. The exact amount of breadcrumbs needed may vary.

4. Divide the mixture into equal portions and shape them into patties.

5. Heat olive oil in a skillet over medium heat. Cook the veggie patties for about 4-5 minutes on each side, or until they are golden brown and heated through.

For Sweet Potato Fries:

1. Preheat the oven to 425°F (220°C).

2. In a bowl, toss the sweet potato fries with olive oil, paprika, salt, and pepper until they are evenly coated.

3. Spread the sweet potato fries in a single layer on a baking sheet.

4. Bake in the preheated oven for about 20-25 minutes, turning them halfway through, until the fries are crispy and golden.

To Assemble:

1. Toast the whole grain burger buns if desired.

2. Place a lettuce leaf on the bottom half of each bun. Top with a veggie burger patty.

3. Add sliced tomatoes and any condiments you like.

4. Place the top half of the bun over the toppings.

5. Serve the veggie burger with sweet potato fries on the side.

Enjoy your homemade veggie burger with nutritious sweet potato fries as a flavorful and satisfying meal! It's a great option for a kidney stone diet, offering plant-based protein and plenty of vegetables.

Roasted Chicken with Rosemary and Garlic

Here's a recipe for Roasted Chicken with Rosemary and Garlic:

Ingredients:

-   4 bone-in, skin-on chicken pieces (such as thighs or drumsticks)

-   2 tablespoons olive oil

-   2 cloves garlic, minced

-   1 tablespoon fresh rosemary leaves, chopped

- Salt and pepper, to taste

- Lemon wedges, for serving

Instructions:

1. Preheat the oven to 400°F (200°C).

2. In a bowl, combine the olive oil, minced garlic, chopped rosemary, salt, and pepper.

3. Pat the chicken pieces dry with paper towels.

4. Rub the olive oil mixture all over the chicken pieces, including under the skin if possible.

5. Place the chicken pieces on a baking sheet or in a roasting pan, skin-side up.

6. Roast the chicken in the preheated oven for about 30-35 minutes, or until the internal temperature reaches 165°F (74°C) and the skin is crispy and golden.

7. About halfway through the cooking time, you can baste the chicken with the pan drippings if desired.

8. Once the chicken is cooked, remove it from the oven and let it rest for a few minutes before serving.

9. Serve the roasted chicken with rosemary and garlic with lemon wedges on the side for a zesty touch.

Enjoy the roasted chicken with rosemary and garlic as a flavorful and satisfying main course. This dish provides lean protein and aromatic flavors that make it a delicious addition to a kidney stone diet.

Spinach and Strawberry Salad

Here's a recipe for a Spinach and Strawberry Salad with Walnuts:

Ingredients:

For the Salad:

- 4 cups baby spinach leaves, washed and dried

- 1 cup strawberries, hulled and sliced

- 1/2 cup chopped walnuts

- 1/4 cup crumbled feta cheese (optional)

For the Dressing:

- 3 tablespoons balsamic vinegar

- 2 tablespoons extra-virgin olive oil

- 1 tablespoon honey or maple syrup

- Salt and pepper, to taste

Instructions:

For the Salad:

1. In a large salad bowl, combine the baby spinach leaves, sliced strawberries, chopped walnuts, and crumbled feta cheese (if using).

2. Toss the salad ingredients gently to mix.

For the Dressing:

1. In a small bowl, whisk together the balsamic vinegar, extra-virgin olive oil, honey or maple syrup, salt, and pepper.

2. Taste the dressing and adjust the sweetness or seasoning if needed.

To Assemble:

1. Drizzle the dressing over the spinach and strawberry salad.

2. Toss the salad gently to coat the ingredients with the dressing.

3. Serve the salad immediately as a refreshing and flavorful side dish.

This spinach and strawberry salad with walnuts is a wonderful option for a kidney stone diet, as it combines nutrient-rich spinach and strawberries with the healthy fats from walnuts. The dressing adds a touch of sweetness and tanginess to enhance the flavors. Enjoy!

Lemon Herb Grilled Chicken:

Ingredients:

- 4 boneless, skinless chicken breasts

- 1/4 cup olive oil

- Juice of 2 lemons

- Zest of 1 lemon

- 2 cloves garlic, minced

- 1 teaspoon dried thyme

- 1 teaspoon dried rosemary

- Salt and pepper, to taste

- Fresh parsley, chopped, for garnish

Instructions:

1. In a bowl, whisk together the olive oil, lemon juice, lemon zest, minced garlic, dried thyme, dried rosemary, salt, and pepper.

2. Place the chicken breasts in a resealable plastic bag or a shallow dish.

3. Pour the marinade over the chicken breasts, making sure they are evenly coated. Seal the bag or cover the dish and refrigerate for at least 30 minutes to marinate. You can marinate them for up to 4 hours for more flavor.

4. Preheat the grill to medium-high heat.

5. Remove the chicken breasts from the marinade and let any excess marinade drip off.

6. Grill the chicken breasts for about 6-8 minutes per side, or until they are cooked through and have grill marks. The internal temperature should reach 165°F (74°C).

7. Remove the chicken from the grill and let it rest for a few minutes before slicing.

8. Sprinkle the grilled chicken with chopped fresh parsley.

9. Serve the lemon herb grilled chicken as a flavorful and protein-rich main dish.

Enjoy the lemon herb grilled chicken as a light and tangy option for a kidney stone diet. The combination of lemon and herbs adds a zesty and aromatic touch to the grilled chicken.

Beet and Goat Cheese Salad

Here's a recipe for a delicious Beet and Goat Cheese Salad:

Ingredients:

- 3-4 medium beets (red, golden, or a mix)

- 4 cups mixed salad greens (such as arugula, spinach, and baby greens)

- 1/2 cup crumbled goat cheese

- 1/4 cup chopped walnuts or candied pecans

- Balsamic vinaigrette dressing

For Balsamic Vinaigrette Dressing:

- 1/4 cup balsamic vinegar

- 1/2 cup extra-virgin olive oil

- 1 teaspoon Dijon mustard

- 1 teaspoon honey

- Salt and pepper, to taste

Instructions:

For Roasting Beets:

1. Preheat the oven to 400°F (200°C).

2. Wash and scrub the beets. Trim off the tops and tails.

3. Wrap each beet individually in aluminum foil and place them on a baking sheet.

4. Roast the beets in the preheated oven for about 45-60 minutes, or until they are tender when pierced with a fork. Cooking time may vary based on the size of the beets.

5. Once the beets are cooked, remove them from the oven and let them cool slightly. Carefully peel off the skin (it should come off easily). Dice the roasted beets into bite-sized pieces.

For Balsamic Vinaigrette Dressing:

1. In a small bowl, whisk together the balsamic vinegar, Dijon mustard, honey, salt, and pepper.

2. While whisking, slowly drizzle in the extra-virgin olive oil until the dressing is emulsified.

For Assembling the Salad:

1. In a large bowl, toss the mixed salad greens with a portion of the balsamic vinaigrette dressing. Adjust the amount of dressing to your preference.

2. Divide the dressed greens among serving plates.

3. Arrange the diced roasted beets, crumbled goat cheese, and chopped walnuts or candied pecans over the salad greens.

4. Drizzle a little more balsamic vinaigrette over the salad if desired.

5. Serve the beet and goat cheese salad as a colorful and flavorful appetizer or side dish.

This salad provides a combination of sweet roasted beets, creamy goat cheese, and crunchy nuts, making it a delightful option for a kidney stone diet. It's rich in vitamins, minerals, and antioxidants. Enjoy!

Tuna Salad with Mixed Greens

Here's a recipe for Tuna Salad with Mixed Greens:

Ingredients:

For the Tuna Salad:

-   1 can (5 oz) tuna, drained and flaked

-   1/4 cup diced celery

-   1/4 cup diced red onion

-   1/4 cup diced cucumber

-   2 tablespoons chopped fresh parsley

- 2 tablespoons plain Greek yogurt or mayonnaise

- 1 teaspoon Dijon mustard

- Juice of 1 lemon

- Salt and pepper, to taste

For the Mixed Greens:

- 4 cups mixed salad greens (such as lettuce, spinach, arugula)

- Cherry tomatoes, halved

- Sliced bell peppers

- Sliced cucumber

- Sliced avocado (optional)

Instructions:

For the Tuna Salad:

1. In a bowl, combine the flaked tuna, diced celery, diced red onion, diced cucumber, chopped fresh parsley, Greek yogurt or mayonnaise, Dijon mustard, and lemon juice.

2. Mix all the ingredients together until well combined.

3. Season the tuna salad with salt and pepper to taste.

For Assembling the Salad:

1. In a large salad bowl, arrange the mixed salad
    greens as the base.

2. Top the greens with cherry tomatoes, sliced bell
    peppers, sliced cucumber, and sliced avocado (if
    using).

3. Spoon the prepared tuna salad over the mixed
    greens and vegetables.

4. Garnish with additional chopped parsley if desired.

5. Serve the tuna salad with mixed greens as a
    nutritious and flavorful mea .

This tuna salad with mixed greens is a wonderful choice
for a kidney stone diet, as it provides a balance of
protein, vegetables, and healthy fats. It's a filling and
satisfying option that can be customized with your
favorite salad ingredients. Enjoy!

Chicken and Vegetable Lettuce Wraps

Here's a recipe for Chicken and Vegetable Lettuce
Wraps:

Ingredients:

For the Chicken Filling:

- 1 pound ground chicken (or turkey)

- 2 tablespoons olive oil

- 1 onion, chopped

- 2 cloves garlic, minced

- 1 red bell pepper, chopped

- 1 carrot, peeled and finely chopped

- 1/2 cup chopped mushrooms

- 1 teaspoon ground ginger

- 1 teaspoon ground cumin

- 1 teaspoon soy sauce or tamari (adjust to taste)

- Salt and pepper, to taste

- Fresh cilantro or green onions for garnish

For Serving:

- Large lettuce leaves (such as iceberg or butter lettuce)

- Hoisin sauce or your favorite dipping sauce

1. In a large skillet or pan, heat the olive oil over medium heat.

2. Add the chopped onion, minced garlic, and ground chicken to the skillet. Cook, breaking up the chicken with a spatula, until it's browned and cooked through.

3. Add the chopped red bell pepper, carrot, and mushrooms to the skillet. Cook for a few minutes until the vegetables start to soften.

4. Stir in the ground ginger, ground cumin, soy sauce or tamari, salt, and pepper. Cook for another 2-3 minutes to let the flavors meld.

5. Taste the chicken filling and adjust the seasonings if needed.

6. Remove the skillet from the heat and stir in chopped fresh cilantro or green onions for added flavor.

7. To serve, spoon a portion of the chicken and vegetable filling onto a large lettuce leaf.

8. Drizzle a little hoisin sauce or your favorite dipping sauce over the filling.

9. Fold the sides of the lettuce leaf over the filling and roll it up like a burrito.

10. Repeat with the remaining ingredients to make more lettuce wraps.

11. Enjoy the flavorful chicken and vegetable lettuce wraps as a satisfying and low-carb meal.

These lettuce wraps are a great choice for a kidney stone diet, providing lean protein and a variety of colorful vegetables. They are also a fun and interactive way to enjoy a healthy and delicious meal.

Quinoa-Stuffed Bell Peppers

Absolutely! Here's a recipe for Quinoa-Stuffed Bell Peppers:

Ingredients:

-   4 large bell peppers (any color)

-   1 cup quinoa, rinsed and drained

-   2 cups vegetable broth or water

-   1 tablespoon olive oil

-   1 small onion, finely chopped

-   2 cloves garlic, minced

- 1 cup diced tomatoes (canned or fresh)

- 1 cup cooked black beans (canned or cooked from dry)

- 1 teaspoon ground cumin

- 1 teaspoon paprika

- Salt and pepper, to taste

- 1 cup shredded cheese (such as cheddar, mozzarella, or a blend)

- Chopped fresh parsley or cilantro, for garnish

Instructions:

1. Preheat the oven to 375°F (190°C).

2. Cut off the tops of the bell peppers and remove the seeds and membranes from inside. Set the bell peppers aside.

3. In a medium saucepan, bring the vegetable broth or water to a boil. Add the quinoa, reduce the heat to low, cover, and let it simmer for about 15-20 minutes, or until the quinoa is cooked and the liquid is absorbed.Fluff the quinoa with a fork.

4. In a large skillet, heat the olive oil over medium heat. Add the chopped onion and sauté for about 2-3 minutes until it becomes translucent.

5. Add the minced garlic and cook for another 1 minute until fragrant.

6. Stir in the diced tomatoes, cooked black beans, ground cumin, paprika, salt, and pepper. Cook for a few more minutes until the mixture is heated through.

7. Combine the cooked quinoa with the black bean mixture in the skillet and stir to combine.

8. Fill each bell pepper with the quinoa and black bean mixture, pressing it down gently to pack it.

9. Place the stuffed bell peppers in a baking dish.

10. Sprinkle shredded cheese over the tops of the stuffed bell peppers.

11. Cover the baking dish with aluminum foil and bake in the preheated oven for about 25-30 minutes, or until the bell peppers are tender.

12. Remove the foil and bake for an additional 5-10 minutes, or until the cheese is melted and bubbly.

13. Garnish the quinoa-stuffed bell peppers with chopped fresh parsley or cilantro before serving.

14. Serve the quinoa-stuffed bell peppers as a hearty and flavorful main dish.

These quinoa-stuffed bell peppers are a nutritious and filling option for a kidney stone diet, offering a balance of protein, whole grains, and vegetables. They are not only delicious but also visually appealing. Enjoy!

Roasted Brussels Sprouts

Here's a recipe for Roasted Brussels Sprouts with Balsamic Glaze:

Ingredients:

- 1 pound Brussels sprouts, trimmed and halved

- 2 tablespoons olive oil

- Salt and pepper, to taste

- 1/4 cup balsamic vinegar

- 1 tablespoon honey or maple syrup

- Optional: grated Parmesan cheese for garnish

Instructions:

1. Preheat the oven to 400°F (200°C).

2. In a bowl, toss the halved Brussels sprouts with olive oil, salt, and pepper until they are well coated.

3. Spread the Brussels sprouts in a single layer on a baking sheet.

4. Roast the Brussels sprouts in the preheated oven for about 20-25 minutes, or until they are golden brown and crispy on the edges. Stir them halfway through to ensure even roasting.

5. While the Brussels sprouts are roasting, prepare the balsamic glaze. In a small saucepan, combine the balsamic vinegar and honey or maple syrup. Bring the mixture to a gentle simmer over medium heat.

6. Let the balsamic mixture simmer for about 5-7 minutes, or until it has reduced and thickened to a glaze-like consistency. Remove it from the heat.

7. Once the Brussels sprouts are done roasting, transfer them to a serving bowl.

8. Drizzle the balsamic glaze over the roasted Brussels sprouts.

9. If desired, sprinkle grated Parmesan cheese over the top for an extra burst of flavor.

10. Toss the Brussels sprouts to coat them with the balsamic glaze and cheese.

11. Serve the roasted Brussels sprouts with balsamic glaze as a delicious and nutritious side dish.

This dish is a great option for a kidney stone diet, as Brussels sprouts are rich in vitamins and minerals while the balsamic glaze adds a delightful tangy sweetness. Enjoy the crispy and flavorful Brussels sprouts as a wonderful addition to your meals.

Green Smoothie with Kale, Banana, and Almond Milk

Here's a recipe for a Green Smoothie with Kale, Banana, and Almond Milk:

Ingredients:

- 1 cup chopped kale leaves, stems removed

- 1 ripe banana, peeled and sliced

- 1 cup unsweetened almond milk (or any milk of your choice)

- 1 tablespoon almond butter or peanut butter (optional)

- 1 tablespoon chia seeds (optional)

- Honey or maple syrup, to taste (optional)

- Ice cubes

1. In a blender, combine the chopped kale leaves, ripe banana slices, unsweetened almond milk, almond butter or peanut butter (if using), and chia seeds (if using).

2. If you prefer a sweeter smoothie, add honey or maple syrup to taste.

3. Add a handful of ice cubes to the blender to make the smoothie cold and refreshing.

4. Blend on high speed until all the ingredients are well combined and the smoothie is smooth and creamy.

5. Taste the smoothie and adjust the sweetness if needed by adding more honey or maple syrup.

6. Pour the green smoothie into glasses.

7. Serve the green smoothie with kale, banana, and almond milk as a nutritious and energizing breakfast or snack.

This green smoothie is an excellent option for a kidney stone diet, as it includes nutrient-rich kale, a good source of vitamins and minerals, and a mix of flavors and textures that make it both delicious and satisfying. Enjoy!

Berry and Yogurt Parfait

Here's a recipe for a Berry and Yogurt Parfait:

Ingredients:

- 1 cup Greek yogurt (plain or vanilla)

- 1 cup mixed berries (such as strawberries, blueberries, raspberries)

- 1/4 cup granola

- 1 tablespoon honey or maple syrup (optional)

- Fresh mint leaves for garnish (optional)

Instructions:

1. In a serving glass or bowl, start by layering a spoonful of Greek yogurt at the bottom.

2. Add a layer of mixed berries on top of the yogurt.

3. Sprinkle a layer of granola over the berries. This adds crunch and texture to the parfait.

4. Repeat the layers until the glass is filled, finishing with a dollop of Greek yogurt on top.

5. If desired, drizzle honey or maple syrup over the top layer of yogurt for a touch of sweetness.

6. Garnish the parfait with fresh mint leaves for a pop of color and freshness.

7. Serve the berry and yogurt parfait immediately as a nutritious and delicious breakfast, snack, or dessert.

This parfait is a great choice for a kidney stone diet, as it combines the protein of Greek yogurt with the antioxidants and vitamins from the mixed berries. The granola provides some healthy carbohydrates and fiber, making it a balanced and satisfying option. Enjoy!

Cauliflower Rice with Black Beans

Here's a recipe for Cauliflower Rice with Black Beans:

Ingredients:

-   1 medium head cauliflower, florets separated

-   1 tablespoon olive oil

-   1 small onion, finely chopped

-   2 cloves garlic, minced

-   1 teaspoon ground cumin

-   1 teaspoon chili powder

-   1 can (15 oz) black beans, drained and rinsed

- Salt and pepper, to taste

- Lime wedges, for serving

- Chopped fresh cilantro, for garnish

Instructions:

1. Using a food processor, pulse the cauliflower florets until they resemble rice-like grains. Alternatively, you can use a box grater to grate the cauliflower.

2. In a large skillet, heat the olive oil over medium heat.

3. Add the finely chopped onion and sauté for about 2-3 minutes until it becomes translucent.

4. Stir in the minced garlic, ground cumin, and chili powder. Cook for another 1 minute until fragrant.

5. Add the riced cauliflower to the skillet and stir to combine with the spices.

6. Cook the cauliflower rice for about 5-7 minutes, stirring occasionally, until it's tender but not overly soft.

7. Stir in the drained and rinsed black beans. Cook for an additional 2-3 minutes to heat the beans.

8. Season the cauliflower rice and black beans with salt and pepper to taste.

9. Squeeze fresh lime juice over the mixture for a burst of citrusy flavor.

10. Garnish the cauliflower rice with chopped fresh cilantro.

11. Serve the cauliflower rice with black beans as a nutritious and flavorful side dish.

This cauliflower rice with black beans is a great choice for a kidney stone diet, as it provides a low-carb alternative to traditional rice and a good amount of fiber and plant-based protein. It's a versatile dish that can be enjoyed on its own or paired with your favorite protein source. Enjoy!

Tofu and Vegetable Kebabs

Here's a recipe for Tofu and Vegetable Kebabs:

Ingredients:

- 1 block (14 oz) extra-firm tofu, pressed and cubed

- 1 red bell pepper, cut into chunks

- 1 yellow bell pepper, cut into chunks

- 1 zucchini, sliced into rounds

- 1 red onion, cut into chunks

- 2 tablespoons olive oil

- 2 tablespoons balsamic vinegar

- 2 cloves garlic, minced

- 1 teaspoon dried thyme

- 1 teaspoon dried oregano

- Salt and pepper, to taste

- Skewers (wooden or metal)

Instructions:

1. If using wooden skewers, soak them in water for about 20-30 minutes to prevent them from burning while grilling.

2. In a bowl, whisk together the olive oil, balsamic vinegar, minced garlic, dried thyme, dried oregano, salt, and pepper to make the marinade.

3. Add the cubed tofu to the marinade and gently toss to coat. Let it marinate for at least 15-20 minutes.

4. Preheat the grill or grill pan over medium-high heat.

5. Assemble the kebabs by threading the marinated tofu, bell pepper chunks, zucchini slices, and red onion chunks onto the skewers in alternating order.

6. Brush the grill grates with a little oil to prevent sticking.

7. Place the assembled kebabs on the grill and cook for about 5-7 minutes on each side, or until the vegetables are charred and the tofu is heated through.

8. Baste the kebabs with any leftover marinade while grilling for extra flavor.

9. Once the kebabs are cooked to your liking, remove them from the grill.

10. Serve the tofu and vegetable kebabs as a tasty and protein-rich main dish.

These tofu and vegetable kebabs are a wonderful option for a kidney stone diet, providing a good source of plant-based protein and a variety of colorful vegetables. They can be served with a side of whole grains or a fresh salad for a balanced and satisfying meal. Enjoy!

Baked Cod with Lemon and Herbs

Here's a recipe for Baked Cod with Lemon and Herbs:

Ingredients:

-   4 cod fillets (about 6 oz each)

-   2 tablespoons olive oil

-   Juice of 1 lemon

-   Zest of 1 lemon

-   2 cloves garlic, minced

-   1 teaspoon dried thyme

-   1 teaspoon dried oregano

-   Salt and pepper, to taste

-   Fresh parsley, chopped, for garnish

Instructions:

1. Preheat the oven to 400°F (200°C).

2. In a small bowl, whisk together the olive oil, lemon juice, lemon zest, minced garlic, dried thyme, dried oregano, salt, and pepper.

3. Place the cod fillets in a baking dish, leaving a little space between each fillet.

4. Pour the lemon and herb mixture over the cod
    fillets, making sure they are evenly coated.

5. Allow the cod to marinate in the lemon and herb
    mixture for about 15-20 minutes.

6. Bake the cod in the preheated oven for about 15-
    20 minutes, or until the fish flakes easily with a
    fork and is opaque in the center.

7. Remove the baking dish from the oven and
    sprinkle the baked cod with chopped fresh parsley.

8. Serve the baked cod with lemon and herbs with
    your choice of side dishes.

Enjoy the baked cod with lemon and herbs as a light and
flavorful main dish. This dish provides lean protein and
a burst of citrusy and herbal flavors that complement
the fish perfectly. It's a wonderful option for a kidney
stone diet.

Spaghetti Squash with Marinara Sauce

Here's a recipe for Spaghetti Squash with Marinara
Sauce:

Ingredients:

-   1 spaghetti squash

-   2 cups marinara sauce (store-bought or homemade)

-   Olive oil

-   Salt and pepper, to taste

-   Grated Parmesan cheese for garnish (optional)

-   Fresh basil leaves for garnish (optional)

Instructions:

1. Preheat the oven to 375°F (190°C).

2. Carefully cut the spaghetti squash in half lengthwise. Use a spoon to scoop out the seeds and stringy center.

3. Brush the cut sides of the spaghetti squash with a little olive oil and season with salt and pepper.

4. Place the squash halves cut-side down on a baking sheet.

5. Roast the spaghetti squash in the preheated oven for about 35-45 minutes, or until the flesh is tender and easily shreds into strands with a fork. Cooking time may vary based on the size of the squash.

6. Once the squash is cooked, remove it from the oven and let it cool slightly.

7. Use a fork to scrape the flesh of the spaghetti squash to create "spaghetti-like" strands. Transfer the strands to a serving bowl.

8. In a separate saucepan, warm the marinara sauce over medium heat until heated through.

9. Pour the warmed marinara sauce over the spaghetti squash strands and toss to coat them evenly.

10. Taste and adjust the seasoning if needed.

11. If desired, sprinkle grated Parmesan cheese over the top and garnish with fresh basil leaves.

12. Serve the spaghetti squash with marinara sauce as a delicious and low-carb alternative to traditional pasta.

This dish is a great choice for a kidney stone diet, as spaghetti squash is low in carbohydrates and provides vitamins and minerals. It's also a satisfying way to enjoy a classic pasta dish while incorporating more vegetables into your meal.

Egg White Omelette with Spinach and Feta

Here's a recipe for an Egg White Omelette with Spinach and Feta:

Ingredients:

- 4 egg whites

- 1 cup fresh spinach leaves

- 1/4 cup crumbled feta cheese

- 1 tablespoon olive oil or cooking spray

- Salt and pepper, to taste

Instructions:

1. In a bowl, whisk the egg whites until they are well combined and slightly frothy.

2. Heat the olive oil in a non-stick skillet over medium heat. Alternatively, you can use cooking spray to coat the skillet.

3. Add the fresh spinach leaves to the skillet and cook for about 1-2 minutes, or until they are wilted.

4. Pour the whisked egg whites over the wilted spinach in the skillet.

5. Allow the egg whites to cook for a few minutes, gently lifting the edges with a spatula to let the uncooked egg flow underneath.

6. Once the egg whites are mostly set but still slightly runny on top, sprinkle the crumbled feta cheese evenly over one half of the omelette.

7. Using the spatula, carefully fold the other half of the omelette over the cheese-covered half.

8. Continue cooking for another 1-2 minutes, until the egg whites are fully set and the cheese is melted.

9. Season the omelette with salt and pepper to taste.

10. Carefully slide the omelette onto a plate.

11. Serve the egg white omelette with spinach and feta as a light and protein-packed breakfast or brunch.

This egg white omelette with spinach and feta is a nutritious and satisfying option for a kidney stone diet. Egg whites provide protein while spinach offers vitamins and minerals. Feta cheese adds a savory touch. Customize with your favorite herbs and enjoy!

Here's a recipe for Grilled Steak with Herb Butter:

Ingredients:

For the Grilled Steak:

- 2 boneless ribeye or New York strip steaks (about 8 oz each)

- Olive oil

- Salt and pepper, to taste

For the Herb Butter:

- 4 tablespoons unsalted butter, softened

- 1 tablespoon chopped fresh herbs (such as parsley, thyme, rosemary)

- 1 clove garlic, minced

- Salt and pepper, to taste

Instructions:

For the Herb Butter:

1. In a bowl, combine the softened butter, chopped fresh herbs, minced garlic, salt, and pepper. Mix well until all the ingredients are incorporated.

2. Place the herb butter mixture on a piece of plastic wrap or parchment paper. Roll it up and twist the ends to create a log shape. Refrigerate the herb butter until it's firm.

For the Grilled Steak:

1. Preheat the grill to high heat.

2. Brush both sides of the steaks with a little olive oil. Season them with salt and pepper.

3. Place the steaks on the grill and cook for about 4-5 minutes on each side for medium-rare, adjusting the time based on your desired level of doneness.

4. Once the steaks are cooked to your preference, remove them from the grill and let them rest for a few minutes before slicing.

5. While the steaks are resting, cut a few slices of the chilled herb butter and place them on top of each steak.

6. The heat of the steak will melt the herb butter, creating a flavorful and aromatic topping.

7. Serve the grilled steak with herb butter as a mouthwatering and indulgent main course.

This grilled steak with herb butter is a delicious option for a kidney stone diet, as it provides high-quality protein and can be paired with a variety of vegetables and salads. The herb butter adds a burst of flavor and richness to the steak, making it a satisfying and flavorful dish.

Broccoli and Almond Stir-Fry

Here's a recipe for Broccoli and Almond Stir-Fry:

Ingredients:

- 2 cups broccoli florets

- 1/2 cup sliced almonds

- 2 tablespoons olive oil

- 2 cloves garlic, minced

- 1 teaspoon fresh ginger, minced

- 1 tablespoon soy sauce (or tamari for gluten-free)

- 1 tablespoon oyster sauce (optional)

- 1 teaspoon sesame oil

- Salt and pepper, to taste

- Red pepper flakes (optional)

- Cooked brown rice or quinoa, for serving

1. In a large skillet or wok, heat the olive oil over medium-high heat.

2. Add the sliced almonds to the skillet and toast them for about 2-3 minutes, stirring frequently, until they are golden brown. Remove the almonds from the skillet and set them aside.

3. In the same skillet, add the minced garlic and minced ginger. Sauté for about 1 minute until fragrant.

4. Add the broccoli florets to the skillet. Stir-fry for about 3-4 minutes, until the broccoli is tender-crisp and bright green.

5. In a small bowl, whisk together the soy sauce, oyster sauce (if using), sesame oil, salt, pepper, and red pepper flakes (if using).

6. Pour the sauce mixture over the cooked broccoli in the skillet. Stir to coat the broccoli evenly with the sauce.

7. Add the toasted sliced almonds back to the skillet and toss to combine.

8. Taste the stir-fry and adjust the seasoning if needed.

9. Remove the skillet from the heat.

10. Serve the broccoli and almond stir-fry over cooked brown rice or quinoa.

11. Enjoy the stir-fry as a flavorful and wholesome meal.

This broccoli and almond stir-fry is a delicious and nutritious option for a kidney stone diet, offering fiber-rich broccoli and healthy fats from almonds. It's a quick and satisfying dish that's perfect for a busy day.

Spinach and Mushroom Frittata

Here's a recipe for Spinach and Mushroom Frittata:

Ingredients:

- 6 large eggs

- 1/2 cup milk or unsweetened almond milk

- Salt and pepper, to taste

- 1 tablespoon olive oil

- 1 cup sliced mushrooms

- 2 cups fresh spinach leaves

- 1/2 onion, chopped

- 1/2 cup shredded cheese (such as cheddar, mozzarella, or feta)

-    Fresh herbs for garnish (such as parsley or chives)

Instructions:

1.   Preheat the oven to 350°F (175°C).

2.   In a bowl, whisk together the eggs, milk, salt, and pepper until well combined.

3.   Heat the olive oil in an oven-safe skillet over medium heat.

4.   Add the chopped onion and sliced mushrooms to the skillet. Sauté for about 5-7 minutes, or until the mushrooms are cooked and the onions are translucent.

5.   Add the fresh spinach leaves to the skillet and cook for an additional 2-3 minutes, or until the spinach wilts.

6.   Spread the cooked vegetables evenly in the skillet.

7.   Pour the whisked egg mixture over the vegetables.

8.   Sprinkle the shredded cheese over the egg and vegetable mixture.

9.   Cook the frittata on the stovetop for about 3-4 minutes, allowing the edges to set.

10. Transfer the skillet to the preheated oven and bake for 15-20 minutes, or until the frittata is set in the center and the top is lightly golden.

11. Once the frittata is cooked, remove it from the oven and let it cool for a few minutes.

12. Garnish the frittata with fresh herbs before slicing and serving.

13. Cut the frittata into wedges and serve it as a delightful and protein-rich breakfast, brunch, or light meal.

This spinach and mushroom frittata is a great option for a kidney stone diet, as it's packed with protein and a variety of vegetables. It's a versatile dish that can be customized with your favorite veggies and herbs. Enjoy!

Grilled Turkey Burgers with Avocado

Here's a recipe for Grilled Turkey Burgers with Avocado:

Ingredients:

For the Turkey Burgers:

- 1 pound ground turkey (preferably lean)

- 1/4 cup finely chopped onion

- 2 cloves garlic, minced

- 1 teaspoon dried oregano

- 1 teaspoon ground cumin

- Salt and pepper, to taste

- Olive oil, for brushing

For Assembling:

- Whole wheat burger buns

- Sliced avocado

- Lettuce leaves

- Tomato slices

- Red onion slices

- Mustard or your favorite burger condiments

Instructions:

For the Turkey Burgers:

1. In a mixing bowl, combine the ground turkey, finely chopped onion, minced garlic, dried oregano, ground cumin, salt, and pepper.

2. Gently mix the ingredients together until they are well combined, being careful not to overwork the mixture.

3.   Divide the turkey mixture into equal portions and shape them into burger patties.

4.   Preheat the grill to medium-high heat.

5.   Brush the grill grates with a little olive oil to prevent sticking.

6.   Place the turkey burger patties on the grill and cook for about 4-5 minutes on each side, or until the burgers are cooked through and have an internal temperature of 165°F (74°C).

For Assembling:

1.   Slice the whole wheat burger buns in half.

2.   Place a cooked turkey burger patty on the bottom half of each bun.

3.   Top the turkey burger with sliced avocado, lettuce leaves, tomato slices, and red onion slices.

4.   Spread your favorite burger condiments (such as mustard) on the top half of the bun.

5.   Place the top half of the bun over the toppings to complete the burger.

6. Serve the grilled turkey burgers with avocado with your choice of side dishes.

Enjoy the grilled turkey burgers with avocado as a lean and flavorful alternative to traditional beef burgers. The addition of avocado adds a creamy and nutritious touch. It's a great option for a kidney stone diet.

classic Greek Salad with Olives and Feta

Here's a recipe for a classic Greek Salad with Olives and Feta:

Ingredients:

- 2 cups chopped romaine lettuce

- 1 cup chopped cucumber

- 1 cup chopped tomatoes

- 1/2 cup chopped red onion

- 1/2 cup Kalamata olives, pitted and halved

- 1/2 cup crumbled feta cheese

- 1/4 cup chopped fresh parsley

- 1/4 cup extra-virgin olive oil

- 2 tablespoons red wine vinegar

-    1 teaspoon dried oregano

-    Salt and pepper, to taste

Instructions:

1. In a large salad bowl, combine the chopped romaine lettuce, cucumber, tomatoes, red onion, Kalamata olives, and crumbled feta cheese.

2. In a small bowl, whisk together the extra-virgin olive oil, red wine vinegar, dried oregano, salt, and pepper to make the dressing.

3. Drizzle the dressing over the salad ingredients.

4. Toss the salad gently to combine all the ingredients and coat them with the dressing.

5. Sprinkle chopped fresh parsley over the top for added freshness and color.

6. Serve the Greek salad as a refreshing and flavorful appetizer or side dish.

This Greek salad with olives and feta is a wonderful choice for a kidney stone diet, as it's rich in vegetables, healthy fats, and a touch of protein from the feta cheese. It's a great way to enjoy a variety of flavors and textures in one dish. Enjoy!

Lentil and Vegetable Soup:

Ingredients:

- 1 cup dried green or brown lentils, rinsed and drained

- 1 tablespoon olive oil

- 1 onion, chopped

- 2 carrots, peeled and chopped

- 2 celery stalks, chopped

- 2 cloves garlic, minced

- 1 teaspoon ground cumin

- 1 teaspoon ground coriander

- 1/2 teaspoon turmeric

- 1/2 teaspoon paprika

- 6 cups vegetable broth

- 2 cups chopped tomatoes (canned or fresh)

- 2 cups chopped spinach or kale

- Salt and pepper, to taste

- Lemon wedges, for serving

- Chopped fresh parsley or cilantro, for garnish

Instructions:

1. In a large pot, heat the olive oil over medium heat.

2. Add the chopped onion, carrots, and celery to the pot. Sauté for about 5-7 minutes, until the vegetables are softened.

3. Stir in the minced garlic, ground cumin, ground coriander, turmeric, and paprika. Cook for another 1-2 minutes until fragrant.

4. Add the rinsed lentils, vegetable broth, and chopped tomatoes to the pot.

5. Bring the soup to a boil, then reduce the heat to low. Cover the pot and let the soup simmer for about 20-25 minutes, or until the lentils are tender.

6. Stir in the chopped spinach or kale and cook for an additional 5 minutes until the greens are wilted.

7. Season the soup with salt and pepper to taste.

8. Ladle the lentil and vegetable soup into bowls.

9. Garnish each bowl with chopped fresh parsley or cilantro.

10. Serve the soup with lemon wedges on the side for a tangy twist.

Enjoy the lentil and vegetable soup as a hearty and nutritious meal. This soup is rich in fiber, plant-based protein, and a variety of vegetables, making it a great option for a kidney stone diet.

Greek Yogurt Parfait with Berries

Here's a simple recipe for a Greek Yogurt Parfait with Berries:

Ingredients:

- 1 cup plain Greek yogurt

- 1 cup mixed berries (such as strawberries, blueberries, raspberries)

- 2 tablespoons honey or maple syrup (optional)

- 1/4 cup granola

- Fresh mint leaves for garnish (optional)

Instructions:

1. In a glass or a bowl, start by layering a spoonful of Greek yogurt at the bottom.

2. Add a layer of mixed berries on top of the yogurt.

3. If desired, drizzle a little honey or maple syrup over the berries for added sweetness.

4. Sprinkle a layer of granola on top of the berries.

5. Repeat the layers until you've used up all the ingredients or reached your desired amount.

6. Finish with a final dollop of Greek yogurt on top.

7. Garnish the Greek yogurt parfait with a few fresh mint leaves for an extra touch of freshness.

8. Serve the parfait immediately as a delicious and nutritious breakfast or snack.

This Greek yogurt parfait with berries is a great option for a kidney stone diet, as it provides protein from the yogurt, antioxidants from the berries, and fiber from the granola. Customize the layers and toppings to your liking for a delightful and satisfying treat.

Roasted Vegetable Medley

Here's a recipe for a Roasted Vegetable Medley:

Ingredients:

- 2 cups mixed vegetables (such as bell peppers, zucchini, carrots, cherry tomatoes, red onion, broccoli florets)

- 2 tablespoons olive oil

- 1 teaspoon dried herbs (such as thyme, rosemary, or Italian seasoning)

- Salt and pepper, to taste

- Grated Parmesan cheese (optional), for garnish

- Fresh herbs (such as parsley or basil), for garnish

Instructions:

1. Preheat the oven to 400°F (200°C).

2. Wash, peel (if necessary), and chop the mixed vegetables into bite-sized pieces.

3. In a bowl, toss the chopped vegetables with olive oil, dried herbs, salt, and pepper until they are well coated.

4. Spread the seasoned vegetables on a baking sheet in a single layer.

5. Roast the vegetables in the preheated oven for about 20-25 minutes, or until they are tender and slightly caramelized. Give them a gentle stir halfway through the roasting time.

6. Once the vegetables are roasted to your liking, remove them from the oven.

7. Transfer the roasted vegetable medley to a serving dish.

8. If desired, sprinkle grated Parmesan cheese over the vegetables for extra flavor.

9. Garnish the roasted vegetable medley with fresh herbs.

10. Serve the roasted vegetable medley as a colorful and nutritious side dish.

This roasted vegetable medley is a fantastic choice for a kidney stone diet, as it offers a variety of vitamins, minerals, and fiber from the mixed vegetables. Customize the vegetable selection and herbs to suit your taste preferences. Enjoy!

CONCLUTON

Kidney stones are typically a painful condition. Fortunately, diet can be an effective tool in managing and preventing kidney stones. Staying hydrated and avoiding certain foods that are high in salt and sugar, and pairing calcium with oxalate rich foods are important elements of a kidney stone diet.